1

PREVIEW

Acute pancreatitis is inflammation of the pancreas that develops quickly. The pancreas is a small organ that plays a crucial role in digestion. Some mild cases of acute pancreatitis resolve without treatment, but severe ones can have potentially fatal complications.

Acute pancreatitis means inflammation of the pancreas that develops quickly. The main symptom is tummy (abdominal) pain. It usually settles in a few days but sometimes it becomes severe and very serious. The most common causes of acute pancreatitis are gallstones and drinking a lot of alcohol.

Table of Contents

ACUTE PANCREATITIS DIET RECIPES

BREAKFAST

1. Herbed Spanish Omelet
Prep Time: 60 minute

240 calories per serving

Ingredients
- 1 lb. potatoes, peeled and diced or shredded
- 2 Tbsp. extra-virgin olive oil
- 1/2 cup diced red onion
- 2 cloves garlic, minced
- 4 large whole eggs, lightly beaten
- 2 egg whites, lightly beaten
- 2 Tbsp. finely chopped fresh parsley
- 2 Tbsp. finely chopped fresh basil and chives
- Salt, to taste
- Sprigs of fresh herbs to garnish (optional)

Instuction
1. In large pan, add potatoes. Cover with water. Bring to a boil and cook uncovered for 3 minutes. Remove from heat. Cover and let stand for about 10 minutes or until potatoes are tender, not mushy. Drain well.
2. In deep 10-inch non-stick skillet, heat oil over medium heat. Add onion and garlic. Cook for about 8 minutes, stirring occasionally. Add potatoes and cook an additional 5 minutes.
3. Combine whole eggs and egg whites. Stir in parsley, basil and chives. Season with salt if desired. Pour mixture over potatoes in hot skillet. Reduce heat and

cook uncovered for about 10 minutes or until bottom
of omelet is golden.
4. If desired, brown top under toaster oven. Garnish
with fresh herb sprigs. Serve immediately.

2. Easy Scalloped Potato White Bean Skillet

Prep Time: 75 minute

420 calories per serving

Ingredients

- 1 Tbsp. extra-virgin olive oil
- 1 medium onion, sliced
- 3 cloves garlic, minced
- 5 ounces mushrooms, sliced
- 2 1/2 cups reduced-fat plant-based half and half (or unsweetened plain milk of choice)
- 2 Tbsp. cornstarch
- 3 Tbsp. nutritional yeast
- 1/4 tsp. nutmeg
- 1/2 tsp. paprika
- 1/2 tsp. ground mustard
- 1/2 tsp. salt
- 1/4 tsp. black pepper
- 6 small (about 4.5 ounces each) potatoes, peeled, thinly sliced
- 1 15-oz. can white beans, rinsed and drained
- 1/4 cup ground cashews
- 1/4 cup fresh parsley, chopped (optional garnish)

Instructions

1. Heat oil in large cast iron skillet over medium heat. Add onion and garlic and sauté for 7 minutes.
2. Add mushrooms and sauté for an additional 2 minutes.
3. While vegetables are sautéing, in a small bowl whisk together half and half (or milk of choice), cornstarch, yeast, nutmeg, paprika, ground mustard, salt and pepper until smooth.

4. Pour sauce into skillet and stir until sauce thickens (about 2 minutes).
5. Preheat oven to 375 degrees F.
6. Add potatoes to skillet and fold into sauce with a spoon.
7. Gently mix in beans until ingredients are well distributed.
8. Remove from stove, cover with foil and place on top rack of oven. Bake for 30 minutes.
9. Remove foil, sprinkle with ground cashews and return to oven. Bake for 15–20 minutes, until potatoes are tender and surface is golden brown.
10. Remove from oven. Garnish with chopped parsley, if using. Serve in skillet.

3. Pistachio Crumble Tacos with Avocado Lime Crema

Prep Time: 40 minute

338 calories per serving

Ingredients
Pistachio Crumble Filling

- 3/4 cup shelled unsalted pistachios, divided
- 1 Tbsp. extra-virgin olive oil
- 1 small red bell pepper, cut into ½-inch dice (about 1 cup; reserve a few tablespoons for the topping)
- 4 ounces button mushrooms, roughly chopped (1¼ cups)
- 1/2 cup onion, finely diced
- 1 garlic clove, minced
- 1 tsp. ground cumin
- 1/2 tsp. dried oregano
- 1/2 tsp. chili powder
- 1/4 tsp. chipotle powder
- kosher salt, to taste
- 8 corn tortillas, warmed

Avocado Lime Crema

- 1/2 ripe avocado, peeled and pitted
- 2 Tbsp. plain reduced-fat Greek yogurt
- Juice of half a lime, about 2 Tbsp.
- 2 Tbsp. chopped pistachio
- 2 Tbsp. fresh cilantro leaves, roughly chopped
- 2 Tbsp. fresh mint leaves, roughly chopped
- 1/8 tsp. kosher salt
- A few pinches chipotle powder

Instructions

1. Place all pistachios in food processor and pulse several times until roughly chopped. Set nuts aside and wipe bowl of food processor clean.
2. Heat oil in large nonstick skillet over medium-high heat. Add bell pepper, mushrooms, onion, garlic, cumin, oregano, chili powder and chipotle powder and cook, stirring frequently, until vegetables are tender, 7 to 8 minutes. (Adjust heat if it's too high.) Stir in 1/2 cup of chopped pistachios, and season with salt, to taste.
3. For crema, place avocado, yogurt, lime juice, 2 Tbsp. chopped pistachios, cilantro, mint, salt and chipotle powder in bowl of food processor. Pulse until all ingredients are well combined. Season to taste with additional salt and chipotle powder, if desired.
4. Top corn tortillas evenly with pistachio filling; top with avocado crema and remaining chopped pistachios. Add optional toppings as desired such as avocado slices, chopped cabbage, diced bell pepper, cilantro and mint leaves, salsa or shredded reduced-fat cheese.

4. Sheet Pan Roasted Vegetables and Beans

Prep Time: 50 minute

270 calories per serving

Ingredients

Vegetable mix:

- 1 small head (about 1 pound) cauliflower, broken into florets
- 1 medium (about 9 ounces) bell pepper, sliced
- 2 small (about 3 ounces each) zucchini, cubed
- 2 medium (about 6 ounces each) sweet potatoes, peeled and cubed
- 1 small red onion, sliced
- 1 15-oz. can white beans, rinsed and, drained

Vinaigrette:

- 2 Tbsp. extra-virgin olive oil
- 1 Tbsp. balsamic vinegar
- 3 cloves garlic, minced
- 1/4 tsp. salt, optional
- 1/2 tsp. black pepper

Topping:

- 1/4 cup chopped fresh parsley
- 1 Tbsp. za'atar

Instructions

1. Preheat oven to 400 F.

2. On baking sheet, arrange vertical rows of cauliflower, bell pepper, zucchini, potatoes, onion and beans.
3. In small dish, mix together olive oil, balsamic vinegar, garlic, salt, if using, and black pepper to make the vinaigrette.
4. Drizzle the vinaigrette evenly over the vegetables.
5. Place baking sheet on top rack of oven and roast until tender and golden, 35-40 minutes.
6. Remove, sprinkle with fresh parsley and za'atar and serve.

5. Sheet-Pan Salmon with Roasted Fall Vegetables
Prep Time: 40 minute

410 calories per serving

Ingredients
- 2 Tbsp. low sodium soy sauce
- 1 Tbsp. sesame oil
- 1 Tbsp. maple syrup
- 1 Tbsp. fresh lime juice
- 1/4 tsp. red pepper flakes
- 1 clove garlic, minced plus 3 whole cloves, smashed
- 2 Tbsp. freshly grated ginger
- 4 5oz. skin-on salmon filets
- 1 small butternut squash, peeled and cubed (around 2 lbs.)
- 1 lb. Brussels sprouts, ends trimmed and halved (or quartered, if large)
- 1 Tbsp. extra-virgin olive oil
- 1/4 tsp. freshly ground black pepper
- 1 tsp. sesame seeds, for garnish

Instructions
1. Preheat oven to 425°F.
2. In baking dish, stir together soy sauce, sesame oil, maple syrup, lime juice, red pepper flakes, 1 clove minced garlic and ginger. Place salmon in marinade, skin side up.
3. Place squash and Brussels sprout in a single layer on baking sheet. Add olive oil and pepper and toss to coat. Place smashed garlic cloves among the vegetables. Roast vegetables for 15 minutes.
4. Remove from oven and stir, pushing vegetables aside in 4 spots to leave openings for each salmon filet. Place

salmon on pan skin side down in the open spaces. Pour
any remaining marinade over salmon and return pan to
oven for another 12 minutes or until salmon flakes
easily with a fork.
5. Garnish salmon with sesame seeds and serve
immediately.

6. Lentil Walnut Bolognese with Spaghetti
Prep Time: 60 minute

460 calories per serving

Ingredients
- 1 cup brown lentils, dried
- 4 cups water
- 1 Tbsp. extra-virgin olive oil
- 1 onion, finely chopped
- 4 cloves garlic, minced
- 2 stalks celery, finely chopped
- 1 medium carrot, finely shredded
- 1/3 cup walnuts, finely chopped
- 1 28-oz. can crushed or diced tomatoes, with juice
- 3 Tbsp. tomato paste
- 1 Tbsp. soy sauce, reduced sodium
- 1/3 cup red wine
- 1 Tbsp. Italian seasoning blend
- 1/2 tsp. black pepper
- 1/4 tsp. salt (optional)
- 12 oz. spaghetti, uncooked
- 1/3 cup chopped fresh basil

Instructions
1. Place Dutch oven or large saucepan on medium heat and add lentils and water to pot. Cover with lid, bring to simmer and cook for 10 minutes.
2. Remove lid and continue to cook lentils for about 2 minutes until almost tender and liquid is absorbed.
3. Add olive oil, onion, garlic, celery, carrot and walnuts. Cook for 5 minutes, stirring frequently.
4. Add tomatoes, tomato paste, soy sauce, red wine, Italian seasoning, black pepper and salt (optional). Stir

well and cover. Simmer for 10-15 minutes, stirring
occasionally, until thickened and vegetables are tender.

5. Meanwhile, cook spaghetti according to package
    instructions until al dente (about 7 minutes). Drain
    spaghetti in colander.

6. Divide spaghetti among 6 serving plates or pasta bowls
    (about 1 ¼ cups each). Top with 1 cup Bolognese sauce.
    Sprinkle with 1 tablespoon chopped basil.

7. Summer Squash Ribbons
Prep Time: 20 minute

110 calories per serving

Ingredients
- 2 Tbsp. extra-virgin olive oil
- 1 Tbsp. fresh lemon juice
- 1 tsp. lemon zest
- 2 Tbsp. coarsely chopped oregano leaves
- 1 Tbsp. chopped fresh thyme
- salt, to taste
- freshly ground black pepper, to taste
- 1/2 small red onion, thinly sliced
- 1 medium-large yellow straightneck summer squash
- 1 medium-large zucchini
- 1/4 cup crumbled reduced-fat feta cheese

Instructions
1. In large bowl, whisk together olive oil, lemon juice, lemon zest, oregano and thyme. Season to taste with salt and pepper. Stir in onion.
2. Cut stem end from squash. Holding stem end of squash and leaning other end on cutting board at an angle, use vegetable peeler to shave squash lengthwise to create ribbons. Stop peeling at seed core.
3. Stack ribbons and cut in half crosswise. Add ribbons to bowl and stir, separating ribbons to cover with dressing.
4. Rotate squash to opposite side and repeat peeling, cutting and mixing with dressing.
5. Peel ribbons from remaining two sides of squash and repeat cutting and mixing with dressing.
6. Repeat with zucchini.

7. Transfer squash salad to serving dish and top with feta. Salad may be chilled and served later in the day.

8. Mushrooms with Apple Herb Stuffing

Prep Time: 55 minute

70 calories per serving

Ingredients
- Canola oil cooking spray
- 20 large button mushrooms, wiped with a damp cloth
- 1 Tbsp. reduced-sodium soy sauce
- 4 tsp. canola oil, divided
- 3 tsp. balsamic vinegar, divided
- 1 small leak, white part only, rinsed and finely diced (about ¾ cup)
- 1 celery rib, minced
- 1 medium red apple, peeled, cored and finely diced
- 2 Tbsp. minced flat leaf parsley
- 1/4 tsp. minced fresh oregano or pinched of dried
- 1/4 tsp. minced fresh basil or pinch of dried
- Salt and pepper, to taste
- 1/2 cup whole-wheat breadcrumbs
- 2 Tbsp. Parmesan cheese, finely grated
- 2 tsp. vegetable broth or water

Instructions
1. Preheat oven to 450 degrees F. Lightly coat baking sheet with canola oil spray.
2. Scoop stems out of mushroom caps with small spoon. Trim and discard bottoms of stems, finely chop stems and set aside.
3. In large bowl, mix soy sauce, 1 tsp. canola oil and 1 tsp. balsamic vinegar. Add mushroom caps. Using your hands or large spoon, toss to coat each mushroom with soy sauce mixture and place, cavity side up, on prepared baking sheet. Set aside.

4. In medium skillet over medium heat, heat 1 tsp. canola oil and sauté mushroom stems, leek, celery, apple, parsley, oregano and basil for 7 minutes, until celery and apple are tender.
5. Remove from heat and season mixture with salt and pepper, to taste. Add breadcrumbs and remaining 2 tsp. canola oil and stir to combine.
6. Transfer mixture to bowl and stir in Parmesan cheese and broth or water. Stuff each mushroom with slightly rounded tablespoon of filling. Brush remaining balsamic vinegar over tops of mushrooms. Bake uncovered for 25 minutes or until mushrooms are tender when pierced with a fork. Serve immediately.

9. Tandoori Chicken Skewers with Mint Raita
Prep Time: 85 minute

220 calories per serving

Ingredients

- 1 cup fat-free Greek yogurt, divided
- 1/3 cup reduced-fat coconut milk, divided
- 2 tsp. curry powder, mild or hot
- 1-2 finely chopped garlic cloves
- 3/4 tsp. sea salt, divided
- 1 Tbsp. canola oil
- 1 lb. skinless and boneless chicken breast
- 12 (8-inch) bamboo skewers
- Canola oil cooking spray
- 2 Tbsp. finely chopped red onion
- 2 Tbsp. chopped fresh mint
- 1 tsp. lime juice

Instructions

1. In wide, shallow bowl or deep plate, combine 2 tbsp. of yogurt with 2 tbsp. of coconut milk, curry powder, garlic and ½ tsp. salt. Mix in oil.
2. Cut chicken lengthwise into 12 strips. Insert skewer into bottom of one chicken strip and work it up lengthwise to top. Repeat with remaining chicken. Place skewers in curry marinade and using your fingers, make sure it coats them. Cover with plastic wrap and refrigerate for 1 to 8 hours.
3. Arrange marinated chicken on paper toweling and blot dry, removing all excess marinade. Heat large skillet over medium-high heat, then coat with cooking spray (Or heat stovetop griddle). Arrange skewers in one layer in pan and cook for 2 minutes, browning chicken. Using

tongs, turn skewers and brown on another side, 2 minutes. Turn chicken and cook until it is opaque and hot around skewer at thickest part of chicken. Transfer skewers to serving plate.

4. While chicken cooks, prepare the raita. In bowl, combine remaining yogurt and coconut milk with onions, mint, lime juice and remaining salt. When possible, make raita 30 minutes before serving chicken to allow its flavors to develop and meld. Serve it the day it is made.

10. Turkey Pot Pie with Cornbread Crust

Prep Time: 80 minute

280 calories per serving

Ingredients

- 1/2 cup sliced carrots, in ½ -inch slices
- 1/2 cup sliced celery, in ½ -inch slices
- 1 cup frozen pearl onions
- 2 cups fat-free, reduced-sodium chicken broth
- 1 Tbsp. extra-virgin olive oil
- 1 1/2 Tbsp. rice flour
- 1 cup reduced fat milk, at room temperature
- 1 tsp. dried thyme
- 2 cups cooked diced turkey breast, in ¾ -inch pieces (see note)
- 1 cup green peas, fresh or frozen
- Salt and freshly ground black pepper, to taste

Topping:

- 5 tsp. unsalted butter
- 3/4 cup reduced fat milk
- 1 large egg
- 1/2 pkg. (10 oz.) cornbread mix

Instructions

1. Preheat oven to 350 degrees F.
2. In medium saucepan, simmer carrots, celery and onions in chicken broth until they are tender, about 5 minutes. With slotted spoon, remove vegetables and set aside. Boil broth until it is reduced to 1 ¼ cups, about 5 minutes. Set broth aside.

3. In heavy saucepan, heat oil over medium heat. Mix in rice flour and whisk constantly for 1 minute as it bubbles. Do not let it color. Slowly add ½ cup of reduced broth and whisk until combined with flour mixture. Gradually add remaining broth while whisking vigorously. Add milk and cook sauce for 5 minutes, whisking often, until it has consistency of light creamed soup. Mix in thyme, turkey, green peas and reserved vegetables. Season filling to taste with salt and pepper. Spread filling in 8-inch square baking dish and set aside.

4. For topping, in microwavable bowl, melt butter. Add milk and egg and mix with fork to beat egg. Stir in cornbread mix. Spoon topping over pot pie filling in baking dish, dropping it in dollops to leave room around edges of pan and between dollops.

5. Bake pot pie for 30-35 minutes, or until topping feels firm to touch, is lightly browned, and filling is bubbling. Let sit for 15 minutes before serving.

11. Tex-Mex Pulled Chicken Sandwich
Prep Time: 375 minute

400 calories per serving

Ingredients
- 1 cup no-salt-added tomato sauce
- 1 Tbsp. no-salt-added tomato paste
- 1 Tbsp. Worcestershire sauce
- 3/4 cup onion, finely chopped
- 3 garlic cloves, finely chopped
- 1-2 canned chipotle peppers, finely chopped
- 1 Tbsp. adobo sauce from canned chipotle pepper
- 2 tsp. ground cumin
- 1/4 tsp. salt
- 1/4 tsp. freshly ground pepper
- 2 lbs. skinless and boneless chicken thighs, fat trimmed
- 2 poblano peppers, halved and seeded
- 1 large onion, halved and cut crosswise into ½ -inch slices
- 6 whole-wheat hamburger buns, split

Instructions
1. In 6 or 8-quart slow cooker, combine tomato sauce, paste, Worcestershire sauce, chopped onion, garlic, chipotle pepper, adobo sauce, cumin, salt and pepper. Spread mixture to cover bottom of cooker.
2. Arrange chicken pieces on top of sauce in cooker. Cover and cook on low for 2 hours.
3. Meanwhile, preheat oven to 450 degrees F.
4. Line baking sheet with foil. Arrange poblano halves skin-side up on baking sheet. Bake until skin is

blistered, 10 to 13 minutes. Wrap peppers in foil and set aside for 5 minutes. With your fingers, pull off skin. Cut peppers lengthwise into ½ -inch strips. Scrub your hands thoroughly.

5. After chicken has cooked for 2 hours, add poblanos and sliced onion to slow cooker, distributing them over chicken. Cover and continue cooking until chicken shreds when picked at with fork, about an additional 4 hours.

6. Remove chicken to plate. One piece at a time, using 2 forks, shred chicken pieces by pulling them apart. Return chicken to slow cooker and mix with sauce, stirring vigorously.

7. To serve, toast buns. For each sandwich, place bottom half of bun on sandwich plate, top with one-sixth of the pulled chicken and cover with bun top. Serve with coleslaw and pickle spears.

12. Vegetable and Lamb Kabobs

Prep Time: 65 minute

420 calories per serving

Ingredients

- 4 wooden or metal skewers
- 1/3 cup finely chopped fresh parsley
- 2 large cloves garlic, minced
- 1 Tbsp. minced fresh marjoram or 1 tsp. dried marjoram
- 1 Tbsp. minced fresh thyme or 1 tsp. dried thyme
- 1/2 cup extra-virgin olive oil
- 1/4 cup fresh lemon juice (about 2-3 medium lemons)
- 1/2 tsp. salt
- 1/4 tsp. freshly ground black pepper
- 1 lb. leg of lamb, fat trimmed and cut in 1-inch chunks
- 1 medium red onion cut into quarters, separated into 8 (2-3-layer) chunks
- 1 large green bell pepper cut into 8 pieces
- 1 medium yellow squash cut into 12 slices
- 8 cherry tomatoes or 1 large tomato cut into 8 wedges
- Canola oil cooking spray

Instructions

1. If using wooden skewers, soak these in water for 10-30 minutes.
2. In mixing bowl, combine parsley, garlic, marjoram, thyme, oil, lemon juice, salt and pepper. Remove ¼ cup marinade, put in small bowl, cover and refrigerate. Use for brushing kabobs while cooking later.
3. To mixing bowl, add lamb and combine with remaining marinade. Cover bowl and refrigerate lamb for a minimum of 30 minutes.

4. On each skewer, arrange 2 chunks onion, 2 pieces bell
   pepper, 3 pieces squash, 2 tomatoes, and 4 pieces lamb
   in desired pattern. For pretty pattern use this order on
   skewer: squash, pepper, lamb, onion, tomato, lamb,
   squash, lamb, tomato, onion, lamb, pepper, squash.
   Discard used lamb marinade. Brush kabobs liberally
   with reserved marinade.
5. If grilling, prepare grill and preheat on medium high. If
   cooking in oven, set top rack to second rung (at least six
   inches from broiler) and turn on broiler. Prepare broiler
   pan with cooking spray.
6. Cook kabobs uncovered 6-8 minutes on each side.
   Before turning, brush kabobs with reserved marinade.
   Use meat thermometer to test for desired doneness:
   medium-rare is 145 degrees F, medium is 160 degrees F
   and well done is 170 degrees F.
7. Serve kabobs with Radish and Cucumber Raita or plain
   Greek yogurt mixed with fresh herbs such as mint or
   dill.

13. Arugula Salad with Kiwi, Strawberries, and Pecans

Prep Time: 20 minute

170 calories per serving

Ingredients

- 1/2 cup orange juice
- 2 Tbsp. honey
- 1 fresh lime juice (lemon may be substituted)
- 1/4 tsp. paprika
- 2 Tbsp. extra virgin olive oil
- Zest of one large orange
- 1 Tbsp. cilantro, finely chopped
- 4 cups baby or regular arugula
- 4 green onions, sliced thin, including green stems
- 4 kiwis, peeled and thinly sliced
- 2 cups strawberries, halved
- 1/3 cup coarsely chopped, toasted pecans
- Salt and freshly ground black pepper, to taste

Instructions

1. In small mixing bowl, whisk together orange juice, honey, lime juice and paprika. When well combined slowly add oil and continue whisking until mixture is smooth. Stir in zest and cilantro. Season to taste with salt and pepper. Set aside and allow dressing to stand for a minimum of 10 minutes for flavors to mingle.
2. On large serving platter or in large salad bowl, spread arugula and sprinkle with green onions. Arrange kiwi and strawberry slices on top.
3. Just before serving drizzle salad with dressing and garnish with pecans.

14. Wild Alaska Pollock Rainbow Bowl with Creamy Green Dressing

Prep Time: 60 minute

710 calories per serving

Ingredients
Dressing
- ⅓ cup mayonnaise
- ⅓ cup plain yogurt
- 2 Tbsp. lime juice
- 1 tsp. honey
- Pinch of black pepper
- 3 Tbsp. water
- 1 packed fresh spinach leaves
- ⅓ cup extra virgin olive oil
- Salt, to taste

Quinoa

- 1 tbsp extra virgin olive oil
- 1 cup quinoa (any variety)
- 2 cups low-sodium chicken broth or water

Vegetables

- ½ lb sugar snap peas, sliced in half on the diagonal
- 12 cherry tomatoes, halved
- 8 radishes, thinly sliced
- ½ cup cilantro leaves
- 2 medium avocados, sliced

Fish

- Cooking spray

- 4 6 oz Alaska pollock fillets
- 2 tbsp olive oil
- 1-2 tsp ancho chili powder, to taste
- Freshly ground black pepper
- 1 lime, cut into 4 wedges

Instructions

1. In a saucepan over medium-high heat, heat oil. Add quinoa. Stir for 5 to 6 minutes, or until the quinoa pops and sizzles and smells toasty.
2. Add broth or water and bring to a boil. Adjust heat to a simmer, cover pot and cook for 15 minutes, or until the water is absorbed and the grains are tender. Fluff with a fork and keep warm.
3. In a blender, combine mayonnaise, yogurt, lime juice, honey, pepper, water and spinach leaves. Purée until smooth. With the blender on, gradually add the oil. Add salt to taste.
4. Bring a saucepan of salted water to a boil. Add snap peas and cook for 2 minutes. Drain in a colander and transfer to a plate. Place tomatoes, radishes, cilantro and avocados on a large plate.
5. Preheat broiler to high and set an oven rack 4 inches below the broiler. Line baking sheet with foil and spray with non-stick spray (Or use non-stick foil).
6. Place Alaska pollock fillets on baking sheet and brush with oil. Sprinkle with chili powder and pepper, and gently rub spices into fish. Squeeze a wedge of lime over each fillet.
7. Broil for 5 to 7 minutes, or until fish is lightly browned and cooked through. Cover loosely with foil and let fish rest for 5 minutes.
8. To assemble, divide quinoa evenly between four bowls. Arrange snap peas, tomatoes, radishes, cilantro and sliced avocado over top. Place Alaska pollock on top and

drizzle with dressing. Serve with extra dressing on the side.

15. Spicy Slow Cooked BBQ Peach Pulled Pork Sandwiches

Prep Time: 495 minute

340 calories per serving

Ingredients

Pulled Pork

- 2.5 lbs boneless pork loin roast (center cut, trimmed of all fat)
- 1 yellow onion, thinly sliced
- 3 cloves garlic, finely chopped
- 2 tsp. apple cider vinegar
- 2 tsp. Hickory liquid smoke
- 1 tsp. salt
- 1 cup homemade spicy peach BBQ sauce
- 8 whole wheat buns

Jalapeño Peach BBQ Sauce

- 1 lb fresh peaches (about 2 medium)
- 3/4 cup sweet onion, chopped
- 1 1/2 Tbsps fresh jalapeño, minced
- 1 Tbsp extra virgin olive oil
- 1/4 cup cider vinegar
- 1/4 cup bourbon
- 2 Tbsp honey
- 2 Tbsp Dijon mustard
- 1/4 tsp chili powder
- 1/2 tsp dry mustard
- 1 Tbsp Worcestershire sauce
- 1/4 tsp salt

Instructions

Pulled Pork

1. Place the sliced onion in the slow cooker and top with pork.
2. Season pork with salt, vinegar, garlic and liquid smoke.
3. Cover and cook on high for 6 hours.
4. Remove pork and transfer onto a large dish; reserve the liquid into a cup and set aside.
5. Shred the pork with two forks and put it back into the slow cooker along with about 3/4 cup of the reserved liquid and 1 cup of the BBQ sauce.
6. Cook on high one more hour.
7. Serve on whole wheat buns.

Jalapeño Peach BBQ Sauce

1. Cut an "X" in bottom of each peach, and blanch in a medium saucepan of boiling water 10 seconds. Transfer peaches to a bowl of ice and cold water and cool. Peel peaches and coarsely chop.
2. Sauté onion, jalapeño, and a pinch of salt in oil in a large saucepan over medium heat, stirring occasionally, until translucent, 8 to 10 minutes.
3. Add peaches and remaining ingredients and simmer, uncovered, stirring occasionally, until peaches are very tender, about 30 minutes.
4. Allow to cool slightly, then puree all ingredients in a blender or food processor to desired consistency.

16. Golden Beet Veggie Balls
Prep Time: 160 minute

280 calories per serving

Ingredients

Veggie Balls

- 1 bunch fresh golden beets (about 5)
- 1 (15-oz) can cannellini beans, rinsed drained (about 1 3/4 cups)
- 2 green onions, diced
- 2 cloves garlic, minced
- 1 cup mushrooms, finely chopped
- 1/2 cup fresh chopped parsley
- 1/2 cup finely chopped hazelnuts
- 1/4 cup ground flax seeds
- 1/2 cup whole wheat breadcrumbs (may use gluten-free)
- 1 tsp. sage
- 1 tsp. tarragon
- 1 tsp. thyme
- 1/2 tsp. smoked paprika
- 1/4 tsp. black pepper
- 2 Tbsp. reduced-sodium soy sauce
- 2 Tbsp. tahini

Almond Sage Crema

- 1 cup peeled, slivered almonds
- 1/3 cup plain, unsweetened plant milk
- 1 Tbsp. lemon juice
- 1 clove garlic
- 1/4 tsp. freshly ground black pepper
- 1/2 tsp. ground sage

- Sea salt (to taste, optional)
- 1 Tbsp. fresh, chopped sage leaves
- 1/4 cup dried cranberries

Instructions

Veggie Balls

1. Trim beets and scrub outside surface, leaving peels on. Shred beets with food processor or box grater.
2. Place beans in a mixing bowl and mash slightly with a potato masher to achieve a thick mixture with some lumps.
3. Add beets, onions, garlic, mushrooms, parsley, hazelnuts, flax seeds, breadcrumbs, sage, tarragon, thyme, smoked paprika, and black pepper. Toss together well.
4. Mix in soy sauce, tahini, and lemon juice—using hands to combine well.
5. Cover and refrigerate for 1 hour (or overnight).
6. Preheat oven to 375 degrees F and spray a baking sheet with non-stick cooking spray.
7. Form 24 golf ball-sized balls out of the mixture and place evenly on baking sheet.
8. Bake veggie balls in top rack of oven for about 40 minutes, until golden brown.
9. Serve with Almond Sage Cranberry Crema.

Almond Sage Crema

1. Soak almonds in water for 2 hours (or overnight).
2. Drain the water and place soaked almonds in the container of a blender or food processor.
3. Add plant milk, lemon juice, garlic, black pepper, and ground sage and process to make a thick, creamy dip.

4. Transfer crema to a dish and stir in fresh sage, cranberries, and salt if desired. May garnish with additional freshly ground black pepper and fresh sage.

17. Roasted Cauliflower with Spiced Tomatoes
Prep Time: 60 minute

100 calories per serving

Ingredients
- 1 tsp. ground cumin
- 1/2 tsp. ground coriander
- 1/4 tsp. ground cardamom
- 1/8 tsp. ground pepper, preferably white
- 2 Tbsp. canola oil, divided
- 7-8 cups medium cauliflower florets (from a 2¼ – 2½ lb. cauliflower head)
- Cooking spray
- 1 Tbsp. finely chopped garlic
- 1 can (8 oz.) tomato sauce, no salt added
- 2 Tbsp. tomato paste
- 2 tsp. raw sugar
- 2 tsp. white distilled vinegar
- 1/8 tsp. ground cloves
- 1/8-1/4 tsp. ground cayenne pepper
- 1/2 tsp. salt

Instructions
1. Preheat the oven to 425 degrees.
2. In a large mixing bowl, combine cumin, coriander, cardamom, ground pepper and 1 tablespoon oil. Add cauliflower and with your hands, toss and rub to coat florets, 1 minute.
3. Line 11-inch x 15-inch jelly roll pan with foil. Coat foil with cooking spray. Arrange seasoned cauliflower in one layer on pan. Bake for 10 minutes. Stir, then bake 10 minutes longer.

4. Meanwhile, in a small saucepan, heat remaining oil over medium-high heat. Add garlic and cook, stirring, until fragrant, 1 minute. Add tomato sauce, tomato paste, sugar, vinegar, cloves, cayenne and salt and mix to combine. Cook until sauce bubbles vigorously around edges of pot.
5. Spoon tomato sauce over cauliflower on pan and mix with spatula until florets are well coated, 1 minute. Roast cauliflower 10 minutes. Stir, and bake until florets are tender, about 5 minutes. Serve hot or warm.

18. Turmeric Broth Detox Soup
Prep Time: 15 Minutes
Serving: 6

Ingredients

FLAVORFUL TURMERIC BROTH

* 1–2 tablespoons olive oil
* 1 onion- diced
* 1 tablespoons fresh ginger, grated or finely minced
* 4–5 garlic cloves- grated or finely minced
* 1–2 teaspoons turmeric powder (or 2–3 teaspoons fresh turmeric, finely grated – or a little of both, see notes)
* ¼ teaspoon mustard seed (optional)
* 1 teaspoon cumin
* 1 teaspoon coriander
* ¾ – 1 teaspoon salt
* 4 cups water
* 4 cups veggie or chicken stock
* ¼ teaspoon cayenne, or more to taste
* Squeeze of lime juice or lemon juice (to taste) or 1-2 teaspoons apple cider vinegar (to taste)

Middle Eastern "Minestrone"

* ½ cup basmati rice (dry) or pasta, quinoa (or 1 1/2 cup cooked)
* ½ cup little dry lentils (or 1 cup cooked)
* 1 cup cooked garbanzo beans (or canned, drained)
* 1 can diced fire roasted tomatoes (or use 1–2 cups fresh, diced tomatoes)
* season with lime and salt to taste, a drizzle of olive oil and fresh cilantro leaves

Chickpea Cauliflower Kale Noodle

- 1– 2 cups cooked chickpeas (or chicken)
- 4 ounces dry noodles (rice noodles are good)
- 1–2 cups chopped cauliflower (optional)
- 2 large handfuls chopped kale
- squeeze of lime

Instructions

1. In a large heavy bottom pot or dutch oven, saute onion in 1-2 T olive oil over medium heat for 5 minutes until fragrant and golden. Add ginger, garlic, and fresh turmeric and saute 2-3 minutes until eh garlic is fragrant and golden. Add the mustard seeds, cumin, coriander, and optional turmeric power and saute 1-2 more minutes.
2. Add water, stock and salt. Bring to a simmer. Add vinegar or citrus. (I like a squeeze of lime) Taste. Adjust salt, lime and spice level to your liking. At this point you will have a flavorful base to add what you like. You can also refrigerate or freeze this in batches for later use.
3. Remember uncooked pasta and beans will double or triple in size, so add moderately (4 ounces dry pasta)
4. Remember to think and be sensible about cooking times for each ingredient you add.

19. Sushi Burrito

Prep Time: 15 Minutes

Serving: 2

Ingredients

- 1 cup sushi rice, rinsed 5 times
- 1 cup water
- 1 tablespoon rice vinegar
- 1 teaspoon sugar
- 1/2 teaspoon salt
- 1 tablespoon mirin
- 1 Sushi Burrito
- 2 nori sheets (seaweed)
- 1 cup cooked sushi rice
- 1–2 teaspoon chili sauce or sriracha sauce
- ½ cup match stick carrots (or strips of cucumber, bell pepper, cabbage or daikon)
- ½ an avocado, sliced
- 3–4 ounces ahi tura, smoked salmon or baked tofu (Trader Joe's Sriracha Baked Tofu is good)
- ¼ cup kimchi (or pickled veggies or pickled ginger)
- ⅛ cup fresh cilantro or scallions
- If you like creaminess, add a squirt of sriracha mayo or this vegan Mexican Chipotle Sauce

Instructions

1. Make rice. Rinse and drain the rice and place in a small pot on the stove with 1 cup water. Bring to a boil over high heat, and immediately cover, then simmer on low heat for 15 minutes. Turn heat off and do not open the lid. Let it sit for 10 minutes.

Place it in a bowl and spread it out. Add the remaining ingredients, gently incorporating with a wood spoon, being careful not to break the rice. Rice is ready when it has cooled to body temperature.

2. Attach two sheets of nori together wetting one inch of one side with water- keeping rough sides up. See photos. You will have one long sheet.

3. Spread 1 cup sushi rice evenly all the way to the side edges, leaving about 1 inch in front. (see photos).

4. Spread rice with the chili paste.

5. Layer carrots, avocado, kimchi (drain it first) , ahi (or alternative), cilantro and the creamy sauce if using, in the center of the rice. Gently roll it up, wetting the last inch of the nori (with water) to seal. Place on a paper towel seam side down. Let sit one minute, then cut in half.

6. If packing for lunch, wrap it up in a paper towel, then wrap in foil or plastic.

20. Spicy Lentil Tahini Wrap
Prep Time: 20 Minutes
Serving: 4

Ingredients

- 1 cup dry lentils
- 1 teaspoon cumin
- 1 teaspoon coriander
- 1 teaspoon olive oil
- salt to taste

Spicy Tahini Sauce:

- 3 Tablespoons tahini paste
- 3 Tablespoons warm water, more to loosen
- 1 tablespoon olive oil
- 2 Tablespoons fresh lemon juice
- 1–2 garlic cloves finely minced
- ½ teaspoon kosher salt
- cracked pepper
- 1 teaspoon sriracha sauce

Wrap ingredients:

- 1 ½ Cups shredded cabbage
- 1 ½ Cups shredded carrots
- 3 C chopped cilantro and scallions
- 2 Tablespoons toasted sunflower (or pumpkin seeds) – optional
- 1 avocado, sliced
- 4 x 12-inch tortillas, warmed

Instructions

1. Cook lentils in a pot of water until cooked al-dente. Drain well and season with cumin, coriander olive oil and salt to taste.
2. While lentils are cooking, make tahini sauce. In a small bowl, using a fork or tiny whisk, mix tahini paste, warm water, olive oil, lemon juice, garlic, salt pepper, and sriracha sauce, until creamy.
3. Prep all veggies.
4. When ready to make wraps, heat tortillas over a gas stovetop, set to medium, flipping and turning frequently until tortillas are warm and pliable, or toast in a toaster oven. Do not over toast, or they will become tough and hard to roll.
5. Divide lentils, cilantro, scallions, and veggies and roll up like a small burrito, Cut in half at a diagonal.
6. Serve with the spicy tahini sauce on the side, spooning it in as you eat.

DINNER

21. Best Ceviche
Prep Time: 15 Minutes
Servings: 6

Ingredients

Ceviche Recipe

- ½ a red onion, thinly sliced, with the grain.
- 1– 1 ½ teaspoon kosher salt, start with 1, add more
  to taste
- ¼ teaspoon black pepper
- ¾ cup fresh lime juice (4–6 limes) freshly squeezed
  (try to use ripe limes)
- 1–2 garlic cloves very finely minced (use a garlic
  press)
- 1 fresh serrano or jalapeño chili pepper seeded
  and very finely chopped. Start conservatively, more
  to taste.
- 1 pound fresh fish- sea bass, red snapper, corvina,
  halibut, dorado, escolar, mahi-mahi, tilapia, or
  hamachi – diced into 1/2 inch cubes.
- ¼–½ cup fresh cilantro, chopped
- 1 cup grape or cherry tomatoes, sliced or cut in half
   (or 1 cup diced tomatoes)
- 1 cup diced cucumber
- 1 tablespoon olive oil (optional)
- optional: 1 semi-firm Avocado, diced, or make
  the Avocado Sauce
- Serve with tortilla chips, or lettuce cups, or see
  more options in the post above.

Optional Avocado sauce:

- ⅔ cup Avocado
- ⅓ cup cilantro
- 2/3 cup water- plus more as needed
- 1 tablespoon olive oil
- ½ teaspoon kosher salt
- 1 teaspoon coriander
- 2 tablespoons lime juice
- 1 garlic clove
- cracked pepper to taste

Instructions

1. Slice the red onion thinly with the grain, and toss in a bowl with 1 teaspoon salt and the lime juice, coating well.
2. Add the fish, garlic and fresh chilies, and gently mix.
3. Add the tomatoes, cucumber, cilantro and olive oil, and give a stir and marinate in the refrigerator for at least 30 minutes before serving (45-60 minutes is ideal). The longer you marinate the firmer and more "cooked" the fish will become.
4. Before serving, taste and adjust the salt and heat. Add more salt or chilies if you like. If adding avocado, gently fold it in right before serving- you may need to add a pinch more salt.
5. To make the optional Avocado Sauce, blend all ingredients in a blender until smooth, adding a bit more water or oil, if needed to get the blades going.

22. Savory Mushroom Crepes with Spaghetti Squash And Sage

Prep Time: 45 Minutes
Servings: 4

Ingredients

Spaghetti Squash Filling:

- 1 smallish spaghetti squash (about 3 pounds)
- 1 tablespoon olive oil
- Kosher salt to taste
- black pepper to taste
- 1/2 onion, diced and sauteed (optional, or sub 1 shallot)
- ½ teaspoon fresh grated nutmeg (or pre-ground)
- 1 tablespoon chopped fresh sage leaves
- 1 teaspoon maple syrup
- 1/2 cup grated Parmigiano-Reggiano or Romano cheese

Crepes:

- 2 large eggs
- ½ cup milk
- ½ cup water
- 1 cup flour
- 2 tablespoons melted butter
- ¼ tsp kosher salt
- Butter, for coating the pan

Mushroom Topping:

- 1 T butter + 1 T olive oil
- 1 shallot, finely sliced

- 8 oz mushrooms- quartered or sliced (cremini, chanterelles, shiitake, morels, porcini)
- salt and pepper to taste
- 1–2 teaspoons chopped sage
- a drizzle of truffle oil– optional

Bechamel Sauce:

- 3 tablespoons butter
- 1/4 cup minced shallots (optional)
- 1/4 cup all-purpose flour
- 2 cups milk
- 1/8 teaspoon ground nutmeg
- 1/2 teaspoon salt

Instructions

1. Start the filling: Heat the oven to 425°F and arrange a rack in the middle. Cut the squash in half lengthwise and scrape out the seeds. Brush the flesh with oil and season generously with salt and pepper. Place the squash halves cut-side down on a baking sheet and roast until fork-tender, about 35-45 minutes. (You could do this ahead.)

2. Make the crepes: In a large mixing bowl, whisk together the flour and the eggs. Gradually add in the milk and water, stirring to combine. Add the salt and melted butter; beat until smooth. Heat a lightly oiled or buttered 8-10 -inch frying pan over medium-high heat. Pour or scoop the batter onto the pan using approximately 1/4 cup for each crepe. Tilt the pan with a circular motion so that

the batter coats the surface evenly. Cook the crepe for about 2 minutes, until the bottom is light brown. Loosen with a spatula, turn and cook the other side. Set aside and stack. (you could make these ahead and refrigerate, covering)

3. Make the Mushroom Topping: Saute the shallot and mushrooms in 1-2 T butter /oil until over medium heat until golden and tender and season with salt and pepper and fresh sage. Drizzle with a teaspoon of truffle oil, if you like. Set aside.

4. Make the Bechamel Sauce. Melt butter in a small, heavy saucepan over medium heat until foaming. Add shallots (if using) and sauté 2 minutes. Do not let brown. Reduce heat to low, add flour, and whisk until smooth and raw taste is cooked off, about 1 minute. Gradually whisk in milk, starting with ½ cup, whisking well, then adding another half cup at a time until all is incorporated. Cook until just thickened, stirring often, about 10 minutes. Stir in nutmeg and salt. Season with ground white pepper. (You could make this ahead, refrigerate, and heat up (whisking) before serving. Loosen, if needed with a little milk or water.)

5. Make the Filling: Remove the squash from the oven and let sit at room temperature until cool enough to handle, about 10 minutes. Scrape the flesh with a fork to make long strands; place in a bowl. You should have about 4 cups. If there is more, save the extra for another use. Add nutmeg, maple syrup, white pepper, sage, sautéed onions (optional) and cheese and mix thoroughly, and

taste for salt, adding more to taste. (You could make this ahead.)

6. Assemble: Divide the squash filling among the crepes, and fold them over. (You could fill these ahead and refrigerate.) Heat ½ T butter and ½ T olive oil in a pan or skillet and fry each stuffed crepe on both sides until golden and crispy, adding more butter if necessary, and placing in a warm oven until all are crisped.

7. To plate, place two crispy crepes on top of each other and cut down the middle, so you have 4 triangles. Stack vertically on a plate and drizzle with béchamel sauce, top with sautéed mushrooms. Serve immediately.

23. Crispy Teff Cakes with Wilted Chard & Fresh Tomato Relish

Prep Time: 5 hours

Serving: 4

Ingredients

- 1 tablespoon olive oil
- 1 shallot, finely chopped
- 2 1/2 cups water or broth
- 1 1/2 cups teff (whole grain, not flour)
- 1 teaspoon salt
- 1 teaspoon Herbs de Provence or Italian seasoning
- 1 teaspoon granulated garlic
- 1 tablespoon olive oil
- 4 cloves garlic, rough chopped
- 1 bunch chard chopped.
- 3 tablespoons white wine
- salt and pepper to taste
- 1 cup cherry tomatoes, halved or sliced
- 1/4 cup Italian parsley (or cilantro or basil) chopped
- 1 tablespoon olive oil
- 1 tablespoon balsamic
- pinch salt and pepper

Instructions

1. In a medium pot, heat oil over medium heat. Add shallot and saute until fragrant and deeply golden. Add water, teff, salt, spices and whisk until smooth. Bring to a boil. Reduce heat to medium-low, cover and cook 15 minutes, or until teff is tender (yet still

intact) and when stirred has a consistency of a thick porridge.

2. Grease an 8×8 inch baking dish with olive oil. Give teff a good stir and pour into the baking dish. Using an oiled spatula, smooth the top. Let this cool and place into the fridge until it sets up and is firm, about 4 hours (or overnight). If making ahead see notes.

3. Once teff is cooled and firm, cut into four squares. Remove cakes, then cut each into two triangles. (See notes, for appetizer version.)

4. Pan fry the teff cakes in a skillet, with a little oil, over medium heat, until crispy and heated through, about 5-6 minutes on each side. Place in a warm oven if you like. (Alternately you can bake these on a greased, parchment-lined sheet pan– 20 mins 400F . Brush the tops with olive oil.)

5. Wipe out the skillet, heat 1 tablespoon oil over medium heat and add garlic, stirring until golden, about 2-3 mintues. Add Kale and gently wilt. Add a splash of white wine and season with salt and pepper. Set aside.

6. Make the tomato relish. Place tomatoes, tparley, olive oil, balsamic in a small bowl and mix. Season with salt and pepper.

7. Assemble: Place the warm, crispy teff cakes (2 triangles per person) on a plate, layering with the chard. Divide the tomato relish over top, spooning any remaining dressing on or around the cakes. Serve immediately!

24. Chicken Tagine with Couscous

Prep Time: 15 Minutes

Serving: 4-6

Ingredients

- 1 1/2 lbs boneless chicken thigh meat (or substitute 3 cups cooked garbanzos, 2 cans drained, or a combination of both. Vegetarians could also add cauliflower.)
- 2 tablespoons olive oil
- Generous pinch salt and chili powder
- 3 medium carrots
- 1 large onion
- 1 tablespoon fresh ginger-minced
- 5 garlic cloves- rough chopped
- 1 teaspoon cumin
- 1 teaspoon coriander
- 1/2 teaspoon ground turmeric
- 3/4 teaspoon cinnamon
- 1/2 teaspoon caraway seeds, optional but very tasty
- 1 teaspoon salt
- 1 teaspoon sugar
- 1 can diced tomatoes (fire-roasted if possible)
- 1/4 cup dried apricots, diced (or sub raisins)
- 1 1/2 cups water
- 1 1/2 cups couscous (or sub 1 cup quinoa)

Green Harissa Sauce:

- 1 cup plain yogurt (don't use zero fat, or if you do, add a tablespoon or two of olive oil) or sub vegan yogurt (like coconut yogurt)
- 1/2–1 bunch Italian parsley, small stems OK (or substitute cilantro)

- 1–2 garlic cloves
- 1/2 to 1 whole jalapeño
- 1/2 teaspoon smoked paprika
- 1 teaspoon coriander (or cumin)
- 1/2 teaspoon salt

Optional garnish: fresh mint leaves, toasted slivered almonds or pine nuts

Instructions

1. Preheat oven to 400F
2. Cut chicken into bigger bite-sized pieces, 1-2 inches, and generously salt and pepper and sprinkle with chili powder (If using chickpeas, see notes).
3. In a large heavy-bottom, ovenproof skillet or dutch oven heat the oil over medium-high heat. Sear chicken a few minutes on each side, until golden brown, turning the heat down to medium if necessary.
4. While chicken is searing, prep the veggies.
5. Slice the carrots at diagonal ⅓ inch thick. Slice the onions into rings ⅓ inch think, then cut into half-moons. Rough chop the garlic, and finely mince the ginger. Chop the apricots.
6. When the chicken is golden, remove it from the pan, and set it aside on a plate (it will finish cooking in the oven).
7. Add the onions and carrots to the same pan (adding a tad more oil if need be) and cook over medium heat for 5-7 minutes, until onions become tender and fragrant.
8. Make a well in the center of the pan, add the garlic and ginger, sauté for 1-2 minutes. Add the spices, and sauté for one minute to bring out their

flavor. Add the salt, sugar, undrained tomatoes, dried apricots and water.

9. Bring to a simmer and stir a bit, scraping up any browned bits. Once it's simmering, stir in the couscous. Nestle in the chicken cover and place in the oven for 15-20 minutes.
10. While it's baking, make the Green Harissa Yogurt Sauce: Place the parsley or cilantro, garlic and jalapeño in a food processor and pulse (or finely chop) then place in a bowl. Stir in yogurt spices & salt.
11. After 15 minutes, pull the pan from the oven. If you want the chicken to darken up a bit, broil for a minute or two. Scatter with the mint leaves, slivered almonds and serve with Green Harissa Yogurt Sauce.

25. Harvest Succotash
Prep Time: 20 minutes

Servings: 6

Ingredients

- 2 tablespoons butter or olive oil
- 1 cup yellow onion, diced
- 4 large garlic cloves, rough chopped
- 1 teaspoon smoked paprika
- 1 1/2 teaspoon coriander
- 1 teaspoon sea salt (adjust to taste- start with less if you know you prefer less salt)
- 1/2 teaspoon cracked pepper
- 2 cups zucchini, diced
- 1 cup fresh green beans, sliced 1/4" inch pieces
- 1 cup okra, sliced (fresh or frozen)
- 2 ears of corn, shucked and kernels removed (about 2 cups), (frozen will work here too)
- 1 cup lima beans
- 1 teaspoon dried basil
- 1/2 teaspoon dried thyme
- 1 cup cherry tomatoes
- 1 handful fresh basil leaves
- 1 tablespoon apple cider vinegar or lemon juice

Instructions

1. Add butter or oil, onion, and garlic to the pan and sauté for about 5 minutes. Add smoked paprika, coriander, pepper and saute another minute.
2. Add zucchini, green beans, okra, and butter beans, plus dried basil and thyme. Sauté 5 minutes over

medium heat. Stir in fresh corn for another 4 minutes or until tender crisp.
3. Add vinegar, adjust salt and pepper. Add tomatoes and basil. Serve.

26. Easy Italian Meatballs
Prep Time: 10 Minutes
Yield:15 Meatballs

Ingredients

- 1/4 cup walnuts lightly toasted and ground (or use a 1/2 cup bread crumbs.
- 1/4 cup fresh parsley, finely chopped
- 2–3 teaspoons mixed fresh rosemary, thyme, and oregano, minced (or 1 teaspoon dried)
- 3/4 teaspoon sea salt
- 1/4 teaspoon black pepper
- 2 large cloves fresh garlic, minced or pressed
- 1 egg
- 1 teaspoon dijon
- 1 pound ground beef
- 1 batch of Fast & Easy Marinara or Simple Oven Roasted Tomato Sauce (or sub 1 jar of store-bought Marinara Sauce)

Instructions

1. Prepare the sauce- Fast & Easy Marinara or Simple Oven Roasted Tomato Sauce.
2. In a bowl mix together walnuts, parsley, rosemary, thyme, salt, pepper, garlic, egg, and dijon.
3. Gently mix in ground beef until just combined. Do not over mix, this can toughen the meat.
4. Roll into balls, a generous 1 oz meatball -yields about 13-16. Pan sear in a preheated skillet over medium-high heat, with just a light coating of oil, until most sides are browned. The goal is just to

brown the outside of the meatballs they will finish cooking as they simmer in the sauce.

5. Place the browned meatballs in the sauce and simmer for about 5 minutes. An instant-read thermometer is helpful here. Internal temperature should be 160 to assure they are done but not overcooked.

6. Serve over pasta, zucchini noodles, roasted spaghetti squash, creamy polenta or tucked into a roll.

27. Thai Basil Chicken
Prep Time: 15 Minutes

Servings: 4

Ingredients

- 3 shallots
- 5 large garlic cloves
- 3–6 Fresno or Thai (spicier!) chilies
- 2 tablespoons avocado oil or peanut oil
- 1 pound ground chicken (or sub ground turkey)
- 1/2 teaspoon black pepper
- 1/2 teaspoon salt
- 2 teaspoons coconut sugar or honey, or sugar
- 1 tablespoon soy sauce or GF Liquid Aminos
- 1 tablespoon fish sauce
- 1 red bell pepper
- 1 cup Thai basil leaves -or Holy Basil (Tulsi) if you can find it, regular basil will work too
- pinch of ground anise seeds if using regular basil (optional)

Instructions

1. If serving with rice, start that first.
2. Heat up a pan or wok to med-high heat. Add oil and shallots, stir for 2 minutes.
3. Add garlic and hot peppers stir for 2 minutes more until shallots are lightly brown on the edges. Scoop out into a bowl and set aside.
4. Without cleaning out the pan, add oil, turn the heat to high, add ground chicken, black pepper, and salt. Stir fry a couple minutes until chicken is cooked and starting to brown. Sprinkle coconut sugar, soy

sauce, fish sauce over the chicken and stir until incorporated. Add the red bell pepper and the shallot mixture. Cook about a minute, just enough to warm. Add basil leaves and turn the heat off.
5. Serve over jasmine rice. Season with more soy sauce if desired.

28. Fresh Summer Corn Chowder with White Fish
Prep Time: 30 Minutes
Servings: 4

Ingredients

- 2 tablespoons olive oil
- 1/2 cup diced white or yellow onion (or sub 1 large shallot)
- 8 ounces new potatoes (new crop yellow potatoes, red, yukon, any with thin skin) – cut into small dice (no bigger than 1/2 inch thick- the smaller you cut them, the faster they will cook)
- 1 ear of fresh corn- kernels sliced off (or 1 1/2 cups frozen)
- 1 cup stock (veggie, chicken or fish) or sub water- or use corn stock (see notes)
- 1/2 teaspoon salt
- Pepper to taste
- 1/8 cup fresh basil leaves – cut into ribbons or torn
- Optional 2–3 tablespoon half and half
- 8 ounces fish- halibut, sea bass, wild Alaskan cod, haddock, salmon, black cod, shrimp, scallops
- olive oil for searing
- salt and pepper to taste

Instructions

1. Heat oil in a large skillet over medium heat. Add onion and sauté until fragrant about 3 minutes. Add potatoes and corn. Saute 2- 3 minutes, add water or stock, salt and pepper and bring to a simmer. Cover, turn the heat down to low and

simmer 10 minutes, or until potatoes are fork-
tender.

2. While the potatoes are simmering, sear the fish.
   Heat oil in another skillet. Season fish with salt and
   pepper and sear each side over medium-high heat.
   Lower heat and cook to your desired doneness. Set
   aside.
3. When the potatoes are fork-tender, uncover and
   cook off a little of the liquid. At this point, you
   could add a few tablespoons half and half or soy
   milk for a little extra creaminess (cook it for a
   minute or two to thicken) or simply leave it out.
4. Stir in half of the basil. Taste, adjust salt.
5. Right before serving, stir in the remaining basil,
   saving a little for the top. Dish up the sweet
   corn"chowder" and top with the seared fish and
   basil.

29. Rustic Eggplant Moussaka

Prep Time: 1 hour
Servings: 8

Ingredients

- 3 lbs Eggplant (2 extra-large or 3 eggplants)
- salt
- 3 tablespoons olive oil or cooking spray

Tomato Meat Sauce:

- 2 tablespoons olive oil
- 1 large onion, diced
- 4 cloves garlic, rough chopped
- 2 lbs ground lamb, ground beef (or use vegetarian ground meat substitute -Gimme Lean or St Ives Meatless Ground.) I prefer lamb.
- 1 ½ cups diced tomatoes, with juices (or 14-ounce can, with juices)
- 3 tablespoons tomato paste
- ½ cup white wine (optional, sub 1/4 cup water)
- 2 teaspoons dried oregano
- 1 tsp sugar
- 1 tsp cinnamon
- 3/4 tsp kosher salt
- 1/2 teaspoon cracked pepper
- 2–3 tablespoons fresh chopped parsley

Bechamel Sauce:

- 3 tablespoons butter or olive oil
- 4 tablespoons flour
- 2 cups milk
- 1/2 tsp nutmeg (use fresh grated if possible)

- 1/4 tsp kosher salt
- 1/8 tsp pepper or white pepper
- 1/4 cup grated Parmesan, Pecorino or Kefalotiri Cheese (plus an additional 1/4 cup for the top-optional)
- 1 egg, room temp, lightly beaten

Instructions

1. Pre-heat oven to 400 F. Cut eggplant into ⅓- ¼ inch thick disks (no thinner), sprinkle with a little kosher salt and let sit in a colander or bowl for 20-60 minutes. Eggplant will start to release liquid (making it less bitter)
2. Rinse well, pat dry and brush each side with olive oil (or use spray oil).
3. Place on a greased sheet pan and roast in a 400 F oven until golden, about 20-30 minutes. Alternatively, you can grill the eggplant on each side (getting nice deep grill marks) then wrapping it in foil after for 10-15 minutes, so it steams and cooks through.
4. While eggplant is roasting -make the tomato- meat sauce: In a large pan, saute diced onion in oil on med-high heat for 3-4 minutes, add garlic, turn heat down to med-low and saute for 8-10 minutes until onions are tender. Add the ground lamb (or beef or vegetarian meat), turn heat up to medium and brown, stirring often, about 15 minutes. Drain fat if any. Add the rest of the ingredients -diced tomatoes, tomato paste, white wine, fresh chopped parsley, sugar, cinnamon, kosher salt and pepper. Stir and cover and let simmer on med-low heat for 20 minutes.
5. Make Bechamel Sauce: In a small pot, heat the butter. Whisk in the flour and let cook for 2-3

minutes on med heat, stirring often. Whisk in the
first cup of milk a little at a time. Whisk well, and
add the 2nd cup. Stirring constantly bring to a boil,
lower heat, and let simmer on low for an additional
2 minutes. Remove from heat and add nutmeg,
cheese, salt, pepper. Set aside to cool. In a separate
bowl, lightly beat an egg, but do not add it just yet.

6. Assemble: Divide eggplant slices into three stacks,
    reserving the best looking largest pieces for the top
    and bottom layers. The others can be placed in the
    middle layer which will be concealed.

7. In a greased 8x 13 inch baking dish, place one layer
    of eggplant. Add half the meat sauce. Add another
    layer of eggplant and the remaining meat sauce.
    Add the third and final layer of eggplant. Whisk in
    2-3 tablespoons of bechamel sauce, into the beaten
    egg (to temper it) then pour this into the bechamel
    sauce, whisking until nice and smooth. Spread the
    bechamel over the final eggplant layer.

8. Sprinkle with the remaining cheese (optional) and
    place in a 350F oven for 50-60 minutes, uncovered
    until beautifully golden. Let stand 10 minutes
    before serving.

30. Japanese Farm-Style Grilled Teriyaki Chicken Bowl

Prep Time: 4 hours
Servings: 3-4

Ingredients

Farm Style Teriyaki:

- 1 pound chicken thighs (boneless skinless) Or sub 4 extra large Portobellos
- 8 ounces shitake mushrooms (optional)
- ¼ cup soy sauce (or use GF Braggs Liquid amino acid)
- ¼ cup mirin
- 1–2 teaspoons grated ginger
- 1 cup rice, rinsed well
- 2 cups water
- Cucumber Ribbon Salad
- 1 large english cucumber
- ¼ cup rice wine vinegar
- 1 teaspoon honey or sugar
- ¼ teaspoon salt
- 1 tablespoon toasted sesame seeds

Garnishes:

- 1–2 avocados (one half, per bowl) , peeled, sliced, salted
- Garnish:
- 1/3 cup chopped scallions (or chives)
- 1 tablespoon toasted sesame seeds

Instructions

1. Place whole chicken thighs in a ziplock bag with soy
    sauce, mirin and ginger and marinate 4 hours or
    overnight. The longer, the more flavor. You could
    add shiitake mushrooms to the same bag if you
    want.
2. After this has marinated, and you are ready to grill,
    cook the rice.
3. Place water and rinsed rice in a medium pot with a
    pinch of salt. Bring to a boil, cover, then simmer on
    low for 20 -40 minutes, depending on rice type (
    read directions) . Leave covered until ready to
    serve.
4. In the mean time, make the cucumber salad
    and preheat the grill to medium high.
5. Cut cucumber in half lengthwise, and scrape out the
    seeds with a spoon. Using a vegetable peeler, or
    sharp cheese slicer or mandolin, peel long thin
    strips or "ribbons" onto a couple of paper towels.
    Blot with a couple more paper towels and place
    them in a bowl. In a small bowl, whisk rice wine
    vinegar, salt and sugar and sesame seeds together
    and pour over cucumber ribbons, toss.
6. Slice the avocado and scallions.
7. Grill the chicken and shiitakes, over medium high
    heat, turning heat down after marking, letting the
    chicken cook through. Move the shiitakes to a
    cooler spot on the grill,or set aside to prevent
    burning.
8. Once cooked through, slice the chicken and
    assemble the bowls:
9. Place rice in the middle, add grilled chicken to one
    side, then avocado, cucumber salad and shiitakes.
    Sprinkle avocado with salt. Scatter bowl

with sesame seeds and scallions, serve with chop sticks.

10. If going vegan, sub 4-5 large portobello mushrooms for the chicken and add 1 tablespoon oil to the marinade and marinate for 1 hour only. To make gluten free, sub GF soy sauce like Braggs.

11. If you can't find toasted sesame seeds, lightly toast raw sesame seeds in a dry skillet until fragrant and golden. They are key.

www.ingramcontent.com/pod-product-compliance
Lightning Source LLC
Chambersburg PA
CBHW051844250726
48659CB00005B/2007